LIFE IN A
STERILE FIELD

John D. Sanidas, M.D., F.A.C.S.

Archway Publishing books may be ordered through booksellers or by contacting:

Archway Publishing
1663 Liberty Drive
Bloomington, IN 47403
www.archwaypublishing.com
844-669-3957

ISBN: 978-1-6657-3922-1 (sc)
ISBN: 978-1-6657-3923-8 (e)

Library of Congress Control Number: 2023903198

Print information available on the last page.

Archway Publishing rev. date: 05/24/2023

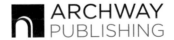

I want to thank all of the patients who allowed me to take care of them for the past four decades.

CONTENTS

OPERATING ROOM

This is always a special room or rooms in a hospital or outpatient surgical facility. The ones in the hospital, of course, where the major surgery is done and contains medical surgical equipment.

The operating room is often on the first floor of the hospital in its own area. This is a clean set of rooms near the emergency room and x-ray department. These entrances are very restricted only to the personnel who work there.

The rooms are clean but can't get completely sterile. That is not quite possible. The sterile part of these rooms are where the surgeon is working. Otherwise the room is as clean as it could be made. It has the usual, necessary, immediate equipment. There are special lights that generally come down from the ceiling that can be operated by sterile handles by the people doing surgery or the circulating nurse. Everyone in the room belongs there.

The door closes itself, which can be entered without any difficulty. This is important for any verbal communication for someone in the hallway or in the area where patients are brought in. Even the phone calls routed through a system are available also to the nurses and doctors in the room.

In addition to the equipment as noted above, we will go into more detail as time goes on. The people in the operating room are wearing special clothing. You cannot go into the operating room with your regular clothes on or even a gown or whatever covering them. You have to go in with the proper wardrobe.

This wardrobe, for all present people in the operating room, consists of a cloth mask to protect the breathing of clean air. This both protects the surgeon from anything, gases coming from the patient itself, protecting the patient from any of the contamination that can occur while talking or expelling saliva, etc., in the operating room.

Clean wardrobe is provided before you go into the operating room for everyone who will be present there. This consists of new, clean that day, pull-over shirt, pants, and also covers for your shoes, so they won't stir up any dirt or contamination from the floor that you would bring in on your shoes. Also, everyone wears a cap or hat to prevent anything from the head and scalp from falling into the wound.

The instructions given to anyone in the operating room: do not reach over the wound unless you have to. Otherwise, you work and use your hands from the sides. Now, it should be also noted that the area sterile is the area prepped for surgery on the patient's body. The room itself is as clean as can be scientifically made. It cannot be completely sterile. The air coming in is filtered air. It is not just plain air.

There are no windows facing the outside of the operating room. There might be windows on the wall of the operating room where students, or people can look in and see what's going on without contaminating the area.

In the operating room, there are special instruments that are available, and always as sterile as we can get them. More sterilized instruments again are always available. The instruments are generally prepared before the patient goes into the operating room.

The operating room table is all metal in order to be cleaned thoroughly. It can be raised, tilted in certain positions automatically. It should be noted that the operating table height is level to the surgeon's comfort and is narrow, so the surgeon can be right against the table, always as sterile as can be, without having to bend or extend his or her back during long surgical cases that might last four hours or more. If there was any bending of the surgeon's back, other than uncomfortable standing, would cause pain. It would cause muscle strain. Therefore, it is a narrow table.

Extensions can be put on the table. The arms have to be spread out and it Is spread out in various attachment for the legs. The table itself can be, parts of it, rolled down or up according to the need.

The operating room staff or the people who have to be in the operating room, although visitors are allowed if they follow all the rules of sterility. Among the permanent personnel that are in the operating room needed for any major surgery consists of the surgeon, his or her assistant, how many or whatever is the need, one or two generally is sufficient. The anesthesiologist who is very important for giving the anesthetic and monitoring the patient's breathing and so forth. The scrub nurse who is at the foot of the table or up over towards the head, depending on the type of surgery being done, who passes the instruments to the surgeon. The surgeon asks the nurse for an instrument and this is passed to him. This is all done very sterile, very professional, no pointed instruments that pointed to either one, and careful not to drop any.

In the operating room, but not necessarily in use at that time but immediately available, are special floor lamps that can be supplemental lights for the surgeon. The surgeon can wear a special headlamp when doing certain surgeries that focus right on the area of the surgery. Often, there are assistants who come in and go or nurses as needed.

The surgeon is in charge in the operating room. As long as the surgeon is there, everything that happens there is under his/her responsibility. The assistant can be a professional assistant that is hired by the hospital or by the doctor to help with the surgery. This assistant also can be a primary doctor who referred this patient to the surgeon. Also a doctor in training, which we call the residents, can be there to help and learn from the surgery. This person doesn't necessarily have to be part of the surgical team, but can observe what is done by looking over the surgeon's shoulder.

The surgeon and his/her assistant and the scrub nurse, and the anesthesiologist, can be in the operating room and have to be in the the clean uniform as described above.

The number of assistants is often decided by the surgeon. Sometimes he or she needs more help with a particularly long drawn out and complicated surgery to have extra people available on as-needed basis. These people don't stay in the operating room. They may be circulating in the operating area until they're called.

An important member of the surgical staff is the anesthesiologist. This is a doctor specialist or nurse specialist putting the patient to sleep safely and have the patient wake up safely. During the surgery, he/she keeps checking the vital signs of the patient and often controls the intravenous fluids, blood, etc., that the patient will need during the operation. The anesthesiologists are trained and experienced enough that they work well with the surgeon, with a dialogue back and forth how the patient's condition is, and where they are in the surgery, and the status, and how much more time is needed.

If there are any complications with what they're doing, they immediately take care and solve any problems that come up. I will take this opportunity to explain that the talking is quite minimal and professional between everyone in the operating room. There is no telling of any jokes which is thought to be a poor form for professional. Occasionally there is music piped into the operating room, which seems to soothe some of the participants and always under the control of the surgeon if it's too loud, etc.

The anesthesiologist also takes care of and is responsible in his area for the patient's vital signs, the oxygen circulation and anesthesia.

Surgery is generalized into two types of surgery, the first being elective surgery, which has been scheduled, planned for a certain date, and the patient is aware what the surgery is being done for.

Emergency surgery is in a separate category. This was not planned for. It's a serious situation, and the patient has been examined in advance probably in the emergency room, and frequently surgery is the answer to the problem. Most hospitals are ready for this type of surgery. Depending on the status of the hospital, it can be categorized whether the hospital can take care of the most major surgeries, or the patient is transferred to the proper facility. This is a type of facility in that the surgeon and anesthesiologist are present in the hospital facility at all times, but exceptions can be made if the surgeon and anesthesiologist live very close to the hospital and can be there within minutes.

In general, this patient is driven to the hospital by a person from family, etc., or brought in by ambulance who knows which hospital to go to or adheres to the patient's choice. They are immediately examined by the emergency room doctor who gets the necessary x-rays and the history and physical. This is all done quickly, but professionally. The emergency room doctor will contact the surgical staff and give them what is the problem and if the patient needs immediate surgery or surgery in the very near future, like in the morning or evening, whichever is available. The surgeon is often in the hospital seeing patients or is close enough to the emergency room that he/she will be there almost immediately to examine the patient also. Then the anesthesiologist is called and everyone meets in the operating room suite area to start doing surgery on the patient.

In general, in an elective surgery, the patient comes in that morning to have the surgery done. Generally, this patient has seen the surgeon in the office preoperatively and is told to come to the hospital at a certain date and time. The patient is then put in the pre-op holding area. This is the area where the patient gets ready for a surgery. The patient is checked over by the nurse, often blood tests or any test can be done on the spot. Occasionally, more x-rays will be needed. However, the patient has been generally worked up thoroughly by the surgeon as an outpatient or in the office.

PRE-OPERATIVE HOLDING

In the pre-op holding, there are nurses there also to evaluate the patient. The patient has most of his or her clothing removed and a surgical gown is put on the patient. Also a label, sort of a wrist band with the patient's name, often the date and the surgeon. That is extremely important for identification because strange as it seems, once people are in bed with a different set of clothing on, they're not easily identified. This is a way of identifying who the patient is and who the doctor is.

The doctor will come in, the anesthesiologist, or both, will come in to check and speak with the patient to find out if he or she is ready for a surgery, and did he or she follow his instructions. In addition to the testing and x-rays, they are told to come to the hospital at a certain time, an hour or two before the surgery is scheduled or more, if that is necessary.

The patient is advised by the staff before the surgery, which is generally the doctor's office, to come to the hospital not eating anything for 8-12 hours, including water. In case, just small sips to take pills. Not to drink anything or eat anything. In other words to come to the hospital "dry and hungry".

The purpose of this "dry and hungry" is extremely important to avoid any vomiting or aspiration. The aspiration can occur if you've had a snack or a full meal, so surgery often has to be delayed later on in the day or even the next day or next week. This is generally the area of the anesthesiologist, but it is so important to avoid this complication that every doctor associated with the patient will ask them that repeatedly.

If the patient has hair in the area of surgery, this is often shaved off, but it is shaved right in the pre-op holding area because that's the way you can keep it clean and not infected. If there are little fine cuts, they will be infected if they had been done 8-12 hours before the surgery. The patient also is advised to take a shower in the morning or evening, whichever is available before he/she comes for the operation, and to wear clean, freshly laundered clothes and to sometimes take little sips of water to swallow their pills. This is again to keep the patients dry and hungry to avoid vomiting, and the vomiting can be aspirated into the lungs and can result in some major complications and infection. This is probably the single most important pre-op order for the patient.

POST-OPERATIVE RECOVERY ROOMS

This is an area where the patient goes immediately after the operation. It is a separate area from the pre-op area, and the patient can be coming out of the anesthesia or still somewhat drowsy following the surgery. Under the instructions of the anesthesiologist, the patient can now be treated by the postoperative staff. This consists of giving medication that's been ordered by the surgeon, keeping them clean and warm and taking their vital signs, which consists of a minimum of the blood pressure, temperature, and lung status.

This is an important area and the patient will often be there for an hour or so. From there, once the vital signs are stable, the patient is taken to his/her room. At that point, the patient should be very well stabilized and awake. If there was a problem in the sense that the patient is having trouble getting awake or having problems of any medical nature, the patient has to go to the Intensive Care Unit (ICU), which is the specialized area for very sick patients and post-op patients where care is taken over and the staff are very specialized in treating any of these postoperative problems that can come up.

This possibility of using post-op recovery and intensive care, the ICU unit, is what the hospital has as compared with the outpatient surgery done in outpatient clinics or facilities. Often, they do not have the facility for keeping the patient overnight or under our observation after a major surgery and that is why it is done in the hospital and not the outpatient facility. Outpatients should be able to leave any time the vital signs are stable, the patient is thoroughly awake, and the surgery is not of a major nature.

Generally, the patient has a family member or friend that will drive them back from the procedure if it's done as an outpatient or more close to a minor surgery, and they do not have to stay in the facility. They're also told not to plan on driving for the rest of the day, even if the surgery is considered minor.

FAMILY DISCUSSIONS

The surgeon generally walks out to the patient's family and explains what what was done. If anything comes up, the patient should stay in the hospital longer or go to the hospital after a minor-type operation. There is facility for keeping the family appraised of the patient condition if it is a long surgery, or there are complications that delay recovery. The staff person might at the desk, taking care of the questions of the family and would always keep them advised how things are going. Often, they will even give information to the patient's family if things are going well, only taking a little longer, etc.

TIMING

The timing of surgery: the patient is always brought into the preoperative holding area, and this takes at least an hour before the surgery. Consequently, it is very important to inform the patient's family if surgery is scheduled for 8:00 A.M., it's closer to 9:00 A.M. when they will be started. There is much to do and must be done preoperatively. That way the family knows that it's an hour late or going to take longer than they thought, if they are apprised of the situation. This information is really important to them.

INTERESTING DETAILS

There are basically two types of surgery, also two ways of doing the surgery. Depending on the organ system, abdominal surgery can be done with open or closed surgery. Open surgery means you have an incision that you use to open and repair or take out or do what is necessary for the surgery. It involves an incision, and then the closure of the incision, where you have sutures or clips to use.

However, since more and more use is found for scopes or laparoscopic surgery, this means you do not need any big incision. A small incision, just in the skin, just so that you can pass this long scope and use other areas to put a scope in, for example abdomen and with an assistant who holds one or two of these scopes, you can do the surgery using this instrument. However, the laparoscopic surgery, like many surgeries that are done closed, is done with a video. It is done with a large screen hooked to a television set in which we can see the pathologies and diseases and work watching them on the screen. Also, you can use the scope, strictly to look through and make a diagnosis of what is wrong.

The question is what basically is the advantage or disadvantage of using the scope surgery and making multiple small incisions in the abdominal wall versus one big incision, which is defined as open surgery. First of all, the laparoscopic surgery has relatively little pain associated with it no matter what was done in the abdominal cavity. The abdomen is in a cavity surrounded by muscles and other tissue, and that has to be pierced with the scope in order to see what the pathology is. The advantage of the scopes are as noted: small incisions. They can be regulated. They are made to be painless by the injection of the small opening with a local anesthetic. Once this is done, the pain is relatively mild when the patient wakes.

We have found that often the organ itself has little or no sensation as far as the pain the patient feels. The patient feels mostly pain from the open incision. It also takes much longer to heal from an open incision compared with smaller scope incisions. This is a significant advantage to patients, which means a shorter recovery time and less use of pain or opioid pills after the surgery.

However, the disadvantage of the scoping is that you have to be extremely careful that you check every quadrant in the abdominal cavity. You do this by doing a superior quadrant and an inferior quadrant as needed. The scope surgery, not only being less painful, requires less time to heal. Small incisions rather than a big one, which is fully deep. There is less chance of any infection. However, there is a disadvantage. If for any reason, with the scope, you see pathology that's too big, for example of the liver, to be brought up from small opening, we can make the opening bigger. Also, if there is a situation of internal bleeding where you cannot get control of the bleeding, the surgeon has the option to open the incision and do an open case of surgery. This should always be in the armamentarium of the surgeon.

Starting a case with a laparoscope is generally explained to the patient that they might wake up with a bigger incision because of things we find or of things we have to have to do. As I noted above, most of the pain is in the incision, not necessarily inside the abdominal cavity. This procedure is advised to be done based on diagnosis. If we see this has to be done open, it just delays the surgery a bit longer. However, it is getting more and more popular among the surgeons, and special training generally is required by using the scope. Consequently, if the surgeon is going to do any operation with scoping, he or she must be trained to open the abdomen. If there is any problems.

In general, there's less blood loss because the incision is smaller. There is probably less chance of infection. However, this is not proven. There is less downtime even from a major operation. You can use a scope now commonly for removing the gall bladder, cholecystectomy. Once all goes well, the patient often can go home later in the day, depending on the opinion and experience of the doctor, or stay in the hospital for a day or more as needed.

However, if the patient was opened up, according to the open form of surgery, he or she will have to spend anywhere from five to seven days or more while healing. It is an advantage to do an operation, if you can and if you have the training and the experience, with the scope.

Once the patient is brought into the operating room, there's a good chance that they will see the instruments being displayed on another table for immediate use as needed for the surgery. These are very shiny. They are clean. They are sterile, and they're under control of what the surgeon wants, and then passed to him by the surgical scrub nurse who is passing instruments.

I'm going to give you a list of surgeries so at least you have a good understanding of what they are and if there are any questions about what they use for. The most instruments will be used when the surgery is an incision. The scope only needs three or four different scopes with lens. Once in surgery, air is used to inflate the intra-abdominal wall so to give space to do the surgery. Once that is done, the scopes come into use. As I said before, you don't need as many instruments when the case is done with the scope. Assisting the scopes will be several different sizes, extra scopes as a standby, and also the open surgery instruments will be available if the type of surgery changes.

For open surgery, there are many impressive instruments. There are mostly metal, and also sponges are used. The patient, of course, can get anxious when he sees these instruments. Remember, they're just there to help you. They don't cause damage in themselves if they are used scientifically.

I will list the instruments with the definition and the use. For example, scissors. They have all sizes of scissors. Some are very long. Some are short. Please note that all of these instruments are made of metal.

We have forceps. Again, all sizes. We have various retractors. These look like bent metal with a handle. These are for opening and keeping the incision open and allowing visibility to the surgeon.

We also have sponge sticks, which hold sponges very tightly in the grasp to sponge and wipe blood away if needed. The sponges we use are cloth sponges. There are various different sizes and are basically cloth towels. Every one of them that we use has a line that can be seen on x-ray. Otherwise, cloth can't be seen on x-ray. This is very important if we want to make sure all the sponges are removed. They will have a metal line to show the doctor if there are any left in the incision and where they are. In addition to the instruments as noted above, we have different splints that can be applied to the appendage, of all types. We have scalpels of all sizes and different blades on them to use.

It is very important that everything we use from the sponges to the instruments that can be shown on an x-ray, prior to the operation, the number of each instrument and sponge is noted by the nurse are recorded and at the end of the surgery, we can always tell by how many we have. We have everything, however, to be double sure and make sure that no small instrument or sponge is left in the abdominal cavity, we take an x-ray. X-ray will help show us when we are finished with the surgery, nothing radiopaque is in there that shouldn't be in there from the surgery. This is very, very important, especially when you have emergency and bleeding situations. We have to act quickly. Now I do emphasize the importance of the counting of the instruments at beginning and end of surgery because the possibility is that one can be left (although rare).

We do call the various incisions for surgery as open and closed. The closed refers to the incision of the area, particularly the abdomen and in the chest, where if it's open, that's a situation where there has to be closure. The closing of the incision can be done with, through the surgeon's judgment, sewing of the different layers of the abdominal wall, including the skin. That is a closed incision. However, if there was a contaminated or an infected area around where the surgery was done, after much irrigation with sterile fluid and cleaning of the area, the surgeon might leave the incision open at the skin level or close very loosely. That is a good judgment in the sense of protection against getting a wound infection.

This is an appropriate time to discuss the complications that can occur with the open surgery, with an incision, or the small opening made with the laparoscope, particularly with the open incision of the abdominal wall and doing the surgery on the organs that you can have postoperative bleeding. That can be anywhere, even in the scope type surgery that can be controlled with clips and cautery (electric current), sutures and various instruments we have. When I say bleeding, I mean bleeding from a removal of an area of the surgery or even a distant organ that can be taken care of immediately by direct vision or opening the incision more or doing another incision.

Therefore, the choice of incision and your choice of the type of surgery, open or close, is a very important decision to make. It takes significant training and experience to decide what is best for the patient. In addition to the bleeding, infection is always a possibility. There are various reasons for infection that the surgeon has no control over, but by using the technique for the open surgery of leaving the skin open, it'll lessen the possibility of getting an infection. We also use drains. These are loose rubber tubes. These are very important because if there is collection of fluid from the surgery or unusual collecting, this can cause some complications, the drains are there to drain out the fluid and you can easily remove them at an appropriate time, and they are safe thing to do so to. You might wake up with some drains, and just remember, that's always there to help the patient.

When all of this is done and the surgery is complete as per the surgeon, the sponge count, instrument count are all correct, a dressing is applied to the incision or to the small opening for the scope. It doesn't have to be a big, giant dressing. It can be a small dressing according to the choice of the surgeon and then held in place with tape, so you do not, in general, leave the operation with just an incision and no covering.

The patient is brought on a gurney, which the patient had been transferred to and wheeled into the recovery room as described above. The final doctor's opinion at that time comes from the anesthesiologist. He stays with the patient until the patient is completely awake and alert and breathing on their own. If there is any question of this, the patient can be given help with the breathing. We have a breathing machine that can be connected to a tube down the patient's throat which can breathe for them. Most of the time that's not necessary, but every so often for a brief time, it is decided by the anesthesiologist otherwise he can leave the postoperative care to the main surgeon and the staff of the recovery room. Generally, by then, the patient is talking, and sometimes complaining of pain for which he/she will be given immediate pain medicine.

If the patient had a major operation, the patient cannot eat or drink anything until the bowels start working again. The patient is nourished and given fluids through the intravenous lines, lines that are generally connected to the extremities. This can last for one day or three, four, five days depending how well the patient does. To feed too early or to give fluids too early by mouth may cause nausea, vomiting, and especially with an open incision, this can be very uncomfortable. This has to be monitored on a daily basis by the surgeon or his assistants.

SURGICAL ASSISTANTS

As I mentioned above, surgical assistants in most major surgeries are judged to be necessary by the surgeon. He/she needs one or two people to assist him with the surgery. This has to be people who are trained to be in the operating room, trained when to assist and sponge the blood away from the wound for the surgeon and to assist in the operation. There are surgical assistants who are trained who will come in and help with most of the cases that the surgeon does. This is particularly true of the open cases as described above. It can involve a regular MD, another surgeon who will assist, or one of these people, or two who are trained as assistants. They are not doctors, but they are very comfortable in the operating room. The main assistant will be the one that helps the surgeon directly.

In the closed scope surgery, the use of assistant is again, up to the surgeon, and this could be one person, generally more. They should be trained in the use of laparoscopic surgery.

ANESTHESIA

There is another form of anesthesia, which is called intravenous sedation and/or local anesthesia with or without IV sedation. This is when a procedure is going to be done, not necessarily a major procedure, but it can be used. For example, removal of a tumor of the hand or abdominal wall where the patient can stay awake and we numb the area of surgery. This is generally a superficial surgery, not in the intra-abdominal cavities. This is done by the anesthesiologist giving the intravenous medication to the patient and the patient goes to sleep. The surgeon also uses a local anesthesia, and this can be done with the patient awakened very easily, right away when we're finished. This is done by neutralizing the intravenous medication by the anesthesiologist. As noted before and I repeat, a significant amount of training and equipment is necessary, but without good anesthesia described above, safe anesthesia, a surgeon cannot proceed and do his part of the operation.

STERILE SURGICAL FIELD

The sterile field, where we all talk about and consider, is the area on the body that the surgeon is operating on. For example, the abdomen, the lower extremities, the chest, and the area he will be operating on is the sterile field. We cannot get a full sterile field because that would cause the skin to be destroyed or irritated. What would happen is it would be an infected area. The sterile field is done by cleaning, washing first with some form of soap and irrigating with sterile water. This takes maybe five or 10 minutes to completely wash it. When that's done, the surgeon will put what he calls paint on this area, which is really a liquid that enhances the sterility. This often contains iodine. This is all done on the skin of the area of surgery. Once we have achieved a significant sterile field, this is blocked off by sterile towels and instruments and the surgery continues. This is a standard procedure for all surgeries. Of course, the surgeon himself or herself has to be as clean as possible. The cleanliness is, again, soap with water. Surgeon washes his hands with free running water thoroughly, and then uses also a brush. The brush has an ordinary part and the other side is a sponge. He can wash thoroughly with the sponge, which has soap inside the sponge, and then clean his nails with the brush. Following this, just irrigate everything thoroughly with clean water as sterile as he can get. The surgeon then dries his hands on a sterile towel given to him by the one of the surgical nurses. Following that, he gets a gown on to protect the patient from anything on his clothing and he is wearing a surgical scrub suit. Once the gown is on and tied from the back, the surgeon has sterile gloves put on his hands by the assistant nurse. This is very important. The gloves protect the surgeon from disease and protect the patient from disease. At the beginning of this procedure, the surgeon has a cap that covers his hair and forehead, and also a mask over his nose and mouth. He can accommodate and talk back and forth without any difficulty and the field is kept sterile as noted above. The idea is to keep the skin clean, close to sterile without injury. But as noted above, you cannot get a hundred percent sterility because that would injure the skin to go so far as to get rid of the bacteria. You get it as clean as you possibly can, and it works very well without any difficulty. The patient, if he is still awake at this time, will see his doctor/surgeon in the full uniform as I've described above.

BECOMING A SURGEON

As we have noted above, we've discussed all the proper techniques and reasons for them for a surgeon to operate. I'm going to go into detail of how you become a surgeon and the type of surgeons there are.

First of all, you must be a medical school graduate of an appropriate school, where you've earned your MD, Doctor of Medicine, or Doctor of Osteopathy, DO. Once this happens, in some circumstances, the doctor has to do another year of training going through the various specialties. However, at the end of getting your degree of medicine, it is noted that you are then a doctor and have to take examinations very soon after for a state license. The license determines your knowledge and training up until then. The internship, which is the rotation when you go through all the specialties, now leads to what's called a residency. A resident means you are a doctor, have a doctor's degree, finished an internship if it's necessary, and have a license to practice medicine in the state where you are taking this training. This training for surgery can be long and it can be difficult physically and mentally, but it has to be done. This consists of four years, in general, to be a general surgeon. That's four years after you have graduated from medical school and after, in some cases, you have finished doing an internship.

The training for a surgeon is one where you are spending most of your time when you're not studying, reviewing, et cetera, medical knowledge with a surgeon, you are now a resident, senior or junior resident or any one through four. You start out by assisting the surgeon in doing the various procedures, and then gradually you go into doing them yourself under the guidance and supervision of the senior surgeon or senior resident. This involves, in most areas, being called at night and operating and doing whatever should be done so that by the fourth year, when you finish your residency, you can be considered a general surgeon and can practice as such. However, you will have to take examinations at the end of that.

Consequently, you go through four years of general surgery training and, if you want to be a specialist on top of this surgery, you have to be a general surgeon first, or take one to two years of the general surgery training to go into orthopedics, gynecology, obstetrics, nose and throat surgery. These are all extra specialties that you can go into once you have your either one or two years of general surgery training, or have to finish and do the four years of surgical training. It's quite long and it will keep you very busy, but we want our surgeons well trained, and this is what they have to do.

Once you have finished all that training that's anywhere from after graduation, medical school of two years, four years or six years, six years, especially if you're going to be a heart surgeon, a vascular surgeon, a pulmonary surgeon, that you must do. Not only are you constantly checked during your training period, but you have to enter the realm of board certification. Board certification has two parts. That's to make sure you've done your training, the training was good, and you know what you're doing and so forth. It consists of two parts of the test generally speaking. The first part is theory, which you fill out the examinations and answer the questions. Following that, and the passage of that, you can practice for two years under supervision or on your own, and then have to repeat examination. That's an oral examination. That means you're sitting down and talking to the senior surgeon or one of the professors and they are giving you instances and what do you do under those circumstances? It should be noted that once you pass the examinations and then you do two years of practice before you do the oral examination, it is a very good idea. That checks even further on the psychology and attitude and reaction with others that the surgeon goes through before he's finally finished, and he must be doing this correctly. Now, once you have passed the oral test in surgery, you are now a surgeon, a full, complete, board certified surgeon, and/or in one of the specialties. Now you continue to do the surgery. You can do it in private practice, join a group, at the university, any number of areas where you can do the surgery, and you are still scrutinized. At this point in time, the surgical examinations, particularly the written, have to be done and renewed every 10 years. In other words, you have 10 years and you must keep up on what's new and what's going on. As long as you practice, you will be required to be take the examination every 10 years. Once you are in practice, the recertification, as it's called, is very important to make sure that the surgeon keeps up on what's new, what's going on, the latest treatments, so it's very safe for the patient. If you are not board certified, generally speaking, you cannot do anything, but the very minor surgery in any hospital.

During all the time of the practice as a surgeon, you will be observed and studied and watched carefully for the safety of the patients. You have to have, in the hospital, attendance at the surgical meetings they have at least once a month, sometimes once a week. In the hospital where you trained or practice or area which you practice will meet for one hour in the morning and go over any surgical business. That includes medicine too, any complaints or whatever. Things like that are very important to your continuing practice.

For example, many institutions, usually the educational ones, have an M and M Conference at least once a week, some longer. The M and M stands for morbidity and mortality, which means complications and problems of the surgery. Mortality, of course, means that the patient died. Any surgeons who have major complications more than the ordinary percentage, or has more death deaths than on the average for the operation will be scrutinized more intensely, and, at the meeting, will explain why a patient developed these complications or death. The discussion will be done in a professional manner of how can one improve. This goes on through the life of the surgeon.

In addition to the above, there are various other meetings that we have during the year (surgery meetings). These meetings will have professors discussing the newest thing in surgery, instruments or whatever. In most states, you have to accumulate a certain number of hours of this per year in order to continue your surgical license. The hours vary anywhere between 20 hours a year and up. This is no choice. We incentivize these people to continue going to school so to speak and continue improving because medicine is a never ending, continuing strive for perfection.

CHECKS AND BALANCES

In order to do the best we can for our patients, there are certain protocols that protect the patient even more than we have discussed up to now. First of all, the importance of the pathologist and the Department of Pathology. No tissue that is removed or organ or problem causing substance that is the reason for the surgery cannot get by without being seen by the pathologist. That means that all tissue removed, gallbladder, appendix, et cetera, must be reviewed by the pathologist. The pathologist is not a surgeon, but he specializes in a micro or macro examination of the tissue. He determines, was it diseased and is the disease now removed? The most common type of procedure with this is a tumor, cancer or otherwise. The tumor is examined by the pathologist and the edges are examined to be sure that everything has been removed. Also, the pathologist not only is necessary after the operation to remove the specimens but during the operation, the surgeon might take what's called a biopsy, small tissue from the tumor or growth, and send it to the Pathology Department while doing the surgery. Pathology will indicate, is this cancerous, or it is not, or whatever it is, and the surgeon will proceed from there with a treatment. Consequently, the pathologist, as noted above, is very important in the cycle of care of a patient.

MORE DISCUSSIONS WITH FAMILIES

There also is another protocol, which we are going to discuss now, that has to be done. It takes information from the surgeon and from the patient. These are questions that you can ask, but generally you don't have to ask many because the doctor/surgeon has a reputation that brought you to go to him/her. Among the many questions, the first one is, "Doctor, what is the diagnosis?" That is the most important in this entire discussion of surgery. Without the correct diagnosis, it becomes difficult or sometimes impossible to tell without the surgery. Most diagnoses can be made before the surgery, but there are times when the patient is acutely ill and you have no time for this and must operate without a specific diagnosis. In any case, any tissue removed, as noted above, is reviewed by the pathologist. The next question is, "What type of surgery are you going to have for your illness?", or "What type of surgery is the surgeon planning for you?" Next question is, "What are the possible complications and the indications for this surgery? Can I postpone it? Do I have to have it now or soon? And what problems can occur?"

The next question is, "What type of anesthesia am I going to have?" There are various statements in this information, which is really a surgical permit, that all patients or family of the patient have to sign. You also can receive a copy by asking for it. Consequently, you have all this information available that is often recorded when you are in the doctor's office, although it can be done before surgery. It is my understanding that this has to be done before you get any sedation to have the surgery, in order that it can be very clear and correct. I'm going to list some tips and some statements that you should keep in mind that you have to have or do before a surgery. We'll take it from the beginning to the end.

MORE TIPS

First of all, you have to be NPO, which is nothing by mouth, before the surgery. In other words, you should be dry and hungry and have nothing to eat or drink eight to 12 hours before the operation (this was noted in the earlier discussion) to avoid any aspiration or throwing up or vomiting or causing problems even before the operation starts. Next, clothes you wear should be clean, laundered clothes, very minimal amount. If you have any jewelry, that should all be taken off also. Next, if you can, take a shower or bath in the morning or evening before the surgery. Any soap will do as long as it is soap, and especially emphasize washing or cleaning the area of your body where the surgeon is going to operate (and-no nail polish or dentures).

You should get to the surgery at least 30 minutes to the time you're supposed to be there. That doesn't mean 30 minutes before the surgery. It's 30 minutes before the time you should arrive. This is very, very important because there is so much to get ready in the surgery, it takes time, and it might run later than you think. This is the opportunity to state, "What difference does it make how long it takes?" Well, it does make a difference, particularly for anesthesia. The longer that they have to keep the patient sedated, the longer it takes for the patient to wake up following the surgery, and also can cause worrying among the people waiting for the final results, thinking that something might have gone wrong. The surgeon should send information back to the family that everything's okay, it's just taking a little longer. As noted, taking longer doesn't mean anything's wrong.

Depending on the surgeon and the anesthesiologist, the anesthesiologist will speak to you very often well before the surgery or at the time of surgery and discuss the medications you are taking, and some you can swallow with a little sip of water or nothing before the surgery is done, but that should be cleared up before the surgery. No creams or ointments should be applied to the area where surgery is going to be done. Just wash with soap and warm water, dry, and leave the rest to the medical staff to do.

It is important to have someone who can drive you back home if this is day surgery done in a day surgery unit. You cannot drive, even though you feel awake and everything is all right, for 24 hours at least following any type of surgery with sedation or otherwise.

SURGICAL AND MEDICAL WOUND CARE

Now that we have reviewed the basics of surgery and some medicine involved, this section will give you more specific cases and the applications of what we have learned from the first study.

Continuing the very important part of this entire discussion is the cleaning of the wound, any wound, small, large, even a deep wound. Also, the wound can be where there is hair and especially in the scalp that's very common. You hit your head, you get a cut in the scalp and you have a laceration. If it bleeds profusely, please note that there's a good vascular supply and the profuse bleeding does not mean it is any more serious than any other laceration. Now, theoretically, you should shave the area of the laceration of the scalp. However, most people do not want that to happen. They want you to suture as is, and you can. You can do this by first cleaning it thoroughly. Again, applying soap, water and good rinsing, good irrigation. Once you do that, you can just suture the laceration and just its surface correction. If it's possible it would be nice to use the suture that is not the same color as the hair. Unfortunately the only color you have is black. Once you suture it, you should leave the sutures long, by that I mean two or three inches, so it can be easily identified when it becomes time to remove the sutures. That removal should be anytime after five days to seven days, and the patient must be warned of being careful when he or she combs and washes the hair. As far as the washing, it can be 24 hours later after the suturing, and they're still careful as noted above. Now, when you get to a deeper laceration, and I'm using the scalp wound as an example since they're deeper, you have to take a curved needle so you can go in deep and sew it shut. We also have staples that can be applied quite easily to the laceration and it does pick up some of the hair but that doesn't seem to be a problem. The staples have to be removed the same way that you remove the sutures. They have a staple remover that works very well.

The question of what type of dressing to put on: that is difficult on the scalp, especially with the hair. There are various dressings, most of them are spray that's actually like a glue or a transparent dressing. I would advise that no dressing be put on. You try to make it as clean and neat as possible. All bleeding should stop. And again you can take these staples out with the staple remover, it's quite a simple technique actually. If there is any question of a tetanus toxoid injection which the patient has not had or did have seven to 10 years ago. According to the clinical determination in the facility where he is, he would have a repeat tetanus toxoid booster or not. That is for the Emergency Room doctor to advise.

Now there is a technical aspect, you have to give some sort of anesthetic because it's too painful not to. That's an injection directly into the wound and on the edge of the wound in about half an inch you inject a small amount. They have many local anesthetics which are available in most emergency rooms. And like I said, that is a judgment call. It's a judgment call for regular lacerations. That type of laceration cut is quite minimal and simpler to take care of. Now why do we go so much into the cleaning and everything? Because if it gets infected then the patient has pain and discomfort, redness and swelling in the area. It often has to be opened with an incision to get the pus out. So the important part here is to make sure you wash it as described.

However, you can note the laceration (cut) can be painful. What we do is numb the area with local anesthetic. The local anesthesia you can use, probably the concentration should be no more than 1% and you can use only so many cc's depending on what local anesthesia you use. You inject it directly into the wound and put as little anesthesia as possible to get slight swelling along the edges of the wound. However, it is not painful anymore and you can do all of these things I described above. That means you do the injection first, numb up the wound and then clean it up as described above. That goes along with all lacerations, especially the contaminated ones that you put on the anesthesia first.

Now as described in this book, the anesthesia is local which is numbing it there, or it can be regional where you make sure you spread out the way you do the injection along the edges of the wound and you try to get any nerves that go there. So to numb it up that way as long as you're under a local anesthetic but be forewarned that these anesthetics are toxic in certain doses so you can't exceed any in these doses. For example, 1% lidocaine injection for local anesthetic cannot go over 10 cc's at a time and preferably below that, and that applies to all local anesthesias. If necessary you could use a general anesthetic if the laceration or the cut is big enough. But then again you have to have an anesthesiologist. You can do it as a regional injection at the base of the finger and inject only medial or inside and outside aspect of the finger. That's fairly far away from the laceration of a finger, even if it's a fingertip but it does numb the entire finger to work on. It should not be used for a rather minor laceration not too large over a centimeter or an inch or so. And even if you have significant bleeding, you could use a tourniquet around the finger. I do not advocate doing that but in some cases you might have to and you should release the tourniquet in no longer than 10 to 15 minutes. If there is enough hair to interfere with your view and whatever of the laceration, that should be shaved off and as I've said before, that should be shaved just before you suture the laceration because it does cause contamination and it should be irrigated thoroughly in case any pieces of hair have ended there.

Now I'm going to get a little more specific. That's the general rule of the anesthesia. Finger cuts are very common. They're common superficial, they're common deep. They can be associated with a crush injury which means the bones could have been involved. And how is that treated? Generally you need to do an anesthetic block at the base of the finger to do the work. So you numb that up thoroughly and then you wash it. Please note this is very important if you don't have to use anesthetic or just small cuts, you can wash it thoroughly and then do needed suturing. You can use skin clips, whichever you're comfortable with. However, when the laceration is very deep, it's right down to the bone or down to a tendon, you numb up the finger, wash it thoroughly after numbing it up and look around if you see a torn tendon. You should close the skin after even more irrigation and send the patient to a hand specialist. Now what you can tell by the examination, if the patient has a tendon cut, is the extension, or flexion. When you ask the patient to extend the finger or flex his finger and he can't then you know you have a tendon cut there. But otherwise in these deep cuts they could have part of the tendon cut and you don't know it-the examination doesn't give you that. So you look down deep into the incision you can spread it over tweezers or tissue retractor and if you see it's cut, the tendon, if it's cut partially and not over 50% of it, you can sometimes just splint it, put it in a splint in flexion after you suture the skin and leave it on for three to six weeks and it can heal. However, I would advise anyone doing that to have a hand specialist do it. It can be quite complicated especially in the fingers. The reason I emphasize this so often is there are so many finger injuries that you see. Those are very common because we use our hands for everything and especially a crushed finger with the bones being fractured, lacerations, that's the problem that has to be corrected in the hospital or in the emergency room.

Now that we have mentioned the splint, that is to keep the finger from either extension or flexion and pulling the sutures out of the tendon or separating it more. When you put on the splint you never put it on the finger straight out because after it's been splinted a while, it can get stiff and you can't bend or move normally. You can avoid most of that by putting the finger or any other joint in a normal position and usually splint it there. There are all sorts of metal splints in the emergency room. And what is the normal position? It is like holding onto a bottle or a pipe or something similar. Just have your hand/ fingers not close tightly, have it around there so you can see the normal use of the hand, how it is at rest, which is around the pipe. Then using that picture in mind, you put a splint on after you suture. The splint, if you have a tendon cut. has to be left on for three weeks or so, but that will be depending on the hand specialist. I do not advise anyone to do this unless you've had the specialty training. Often the cut or bruise can be associated with a bone injury or a nerve injury and the only way really to tell if the bone is involved is to x-ray and you should x-ray it before you suture it. But after you clean it. Don't send them to the x-ray job department with a bleeding dirty wound, you don't know how long it'll take. So clean it good, put a dressing over it, the dressing can be anything that works: a small or large bandaid or sterile four by four put on the wound and then taped in place. Anything that can be comfortably done, then you send them to x-ray. Do not send the patient to x-ray with the wound just open without any treatment or dressing or that will only contaminate it more. If this x-ray shows a fracture and whatever is lacerated at the ankle, the foot, the hand, this is considered an open fracture. That is the definition, that is correct. And the difference is that open fractures when they're superficial and small, they don't require any more cares as noted above. However, when you get into a deep laceration or it goes down to the bone or down to the muscle, particularly the extremities, then it becomes much more serious but it'll need, with a fracture, it'll need a splint in addition to everything else you're doing. So that should be done in a hospital in the emergency room or in the operating room depending on what the surgeon wants to do with the patient and how to help him. It goes for all lacerations, particularly of the extremities. The laceration of the abdomen, a deep stab wound or gunshot wound or whatever needs to be taken care of as soon as possible by a specialist and the wound can just be covered because the patient's going to have surgery and closing will be done under anesthesia.

I will discuss the complications of the infection as noted above, it's a red, swollen wound and can contain pus and be very painful. That's a generic wound infection and if it's of any extremity and it was a superficial or not too deep type laceration, you just open up the incision. You have to get it clean air because the bacteria that cause the infection like dark, moist places. Please note that the dark moist places in the skin or anywhere because that they just thrive on it. But if you take the sutures out or even have to reopen the incision, you clean it out, thoroughly wash it, use just soap water and leave it open. You do not sew it closed. Now the wound will close itself as if it's not infected. It will be slow, and need dressing changes maybe every day and a little more washing off and on, but it will close if the infection is under control.

This is where an antibiotic would come in handy. The minute you suspect it's infected and especially noted with pus and redness and everything, you should give an antibiotic in addition to the situation, we get to wash it open it and so forth. Now what happens to this, if it doesn't heal? If it's an extremity, you'll see the redness, the swelling and you would see, they call red streaks, which are really lymph lymphs tissue and with lymph nodes in the elbow and in the armpit, and it would stop swelling in there and the wound is spread more. This can be a very serious situation needing IV antibiotics. And what's the worst outcome? The worst outcome is that you have an amputation to do, which has to be left open or the patient could be terribly sick, can be awfully sick and die. It's called sepsis. That means the infection has gone into the bloodstream and is being distributed everywhere in the body, and even a brain abcess and death.

Now that is an extreme case that I've just described. And really is quite rare because of the people who know how to take care of wounds and so forth. It's not given to scare you, but given to your thought process. So you'll always keep that in mind. That it's worth the time to examine it and to clean it thoroughly. No matter what it is, how superficial it is, it can go on and cause actually death by septicemia, which means that the bacteria is all over in the blood system. Again, this is rather rare in a civilian treatment, civilian population, but it is always possible and good to know to how to avoid it.

Now I have given you a rather mild minimal cut compared to a serious major cut. The two are very distinctive and one just has to be careful and keep that in mind. Also could be associated with this injury that causes a small laceration or a bump or a bruise and some swelling immediately, which is some blood being in under the wound that accumulated some blood and it causes a little mild discomfort there. Leave it alone. If it doesn't get infected, it will be absorbed. And if the job is done well and the preparation, it will go away by itself, absorbed.

Now continuing on to the major injuries and going a bit in the area of trauma. You have certain rules that differentiate trauma from the ordinary civilian injury and the main difference now I will describe. In the civilian population, these injuries can occur by accident, by not being careful, or a motor vehicle accident. They can have a cut bruise and have a head injury, even though it doesn't look like much. A small cut, there can be a head injury. You don't have to have the injury to the head directly to have a hemorrhage in the brain. I mentioned this because of the seriousness. If the patient complains of a headache and has had a laceration in their scalp, that's not too conclusive for something bad. But if they are getting dizzy, nauseated, cannot see properly, cannot think properly, double vision, then we have a more serious situation on our hands. In that situation, we get a consultation with a specialist, neurologist or a surgeon to get various x-rays, CAT scans, MRIs of the brain for example. The patient has to be under observation in the hospital. That is generally rather common with what they call a neck sprain because in the injury with the car you see the head can project backwards and then when the car stops it can project forward and the brain is not hit, the head is not injured even at all, but the symptoms prevail. The best way to consider this is to think of the brain in a bowl of jelly, attached to the wall with jelly strings. When you do this forward and backward motion, which is called whiplash, the brain is pulled. Even though no injury to the head, the brain can be pulled forward and then back in a closed environment and be injured.

Now this is what is seen in most civilian accidents, motor vehicle accidents, falling and so forth. And they can be treated easily and recognized in the hospital. However, in the military situation, and I do want to mention this briefly, the difference between injuries in the military as compared to the civilian. If it's a serious injury, generally it's more serious because the common cause of deaths in the military are exsanguination, which is bleeding, hemorrhage, loss of blood. And that occurs because the explosives that we use and the various weapons are to cause as much injury as possible in the person. Therefore, if someone has been shot by a bullet or cut by a knife or a fall, you have to be especially careful and have some extra training actually and in trauma in the military situation. I will not go into detail of this, as it is beyond the necessity of this discussion, but it is a good thing to remember that there was a difference between the two.

There are many other situations as described above, but this is the basics of how to treat them, the importance of the diagnosis, how deep is the injury and contaminated in other portion of the injury, tendons and nerves, bleeding et cetera, are they injured.

Because the fingers on the hand are so commonly injured, I do recommend that if you have a laceration deep or superficial, you just put it next to the other finger and bend it. And if it bends the same with minimal discomfort and it can be and extended and flexed, it's a good sign that there's no tendon injury. However, also check the sensation of the finger, both on the inside and outside, just running your hand fingering, comparing the two. Does this feel the same with this? If the patient says it's slightly different on the injured side that I would not get too concerned about that. It is probably due to the laceration swelling. However, if it is completely numb or near, completely numb, when the patient does not feel anything, that might be a signal of a cut, injured nerve, it should be noted. Go ahead and suture it and send it immediately to the hand surgeon.

All the above are very important. And if I stated the basic way of treatment again, because in the civilian world the injuries particularly are of the hand. In the military situation it is quite different. The basics are quite different and you can find information by looking it up on what to do.

So to summarize, the medical problem or injury should be corrected when the patient stabilizes, if there was time with the end of surgery. If this is not an emergency. And any brain surgery, of course, except for the acute ones where injury and blood accumulating in the skull, in the brain cavity, generally speaking, we have enough CAT scans and MRIs to make this diagnosis satisfactory and treat it.

I should mention the great importance of the patient's vital signs, particularly the patient's blood pressure, because during the surgery and the length of the surgery, what it's for, if the patient develops hypertension, or high blood pressure, this must be immediately noted by the anesthesiologist and medication given to lower the patient's blood pressure. If it continues to be observed or continues to go up, a patient can have a stroke or bleed in the skull, in the brain cavity, and this would cause endless complications. So it is very important, particularly if the patient has been taking pills and treated for this by his doctor. Quite simply, just taking the pill before the surgery with a tiny sip of water is perfectly appropriate.

As I had mentioned previously, the importance of avoiding or treating brain injuries. I should also mention that it is the anesthesia and the surgeon's obligation to have the patient in a comfortable procedure to have surgery. Most surgeries can be done with a patient laying on his or her back with the arms outstretched for IV fluids if necessary. This is important because a patient is completely under our responsible control. Not putting the arm in a good position, or injuring the feet, or stretching the extremities can cause injury to the patient because they're completely asleep with the anesthesia as a guide. Therefore, we have various positions and equipment that we can position the patient on his or her side, on the abdomen, or the back. But all of these are used because a patient, as noted above, is our total responsibility. All surgeons have seen a temporary paralysis or pain down a patient's extremity because of stretching or pulling not appropriately or too hard during surgery or in the pre-op preparation. Consequently, this is extremely important, and protocol must be followed.

I do repeat that the surgery with medical problems were coordinated and treated by both physicians (surgeons and primary doctor), and this is very appropriate and the way to do it before, during and after surgery.

DERMATOLOGY

With more and more people enjoying the summer and the sun and the sports in the sun, are prone to skin cancer. These are treated by a dermatologist. The types that I present here are very common and the symptoms are quite similar. They are the melanoma, squamous cell carcinoma, and basal cell carcinoma. They are all basically similar but have serious differences. I will describe in detail the generic transformation or changes that you see in the mole that is consistent with other skin lesions that become cancerous. The melanoma is a cancer from a mole.

The mole ordinarily is normal in color in the sense that it's all a light, smooth brown color. It has no irregularities around the edges, and has no defects or changes in the body itself. Just remember the first important thing in having a suspicious skin lesion is any change. If it was looking one way and they start changing with any of the above, one is concerned and should see the dermatologist. That also applies to skin lesions that start bleeding, minimum amounts that they didn't do before, and slow healing of any lesion. Any cut or any pimple that has slow healing or delayed healing is very suspicious. Now, relatively little pain and the above are generic for having a skin cancer.

Now the melanoma, which is one of the most common, comes from a mole. The mole starts itching, seems to change in color from light, smooth brown to brown spots or any irregular color. The edges of the mole get irregular and at a slight touch it might bleed, and it does appear to be thicker. Again, this description will fit most skin lesions, even those that are not melanomas.

The other cancers, the squamous cell carcinoma and the basal cell carcinoma are in skin lesions that will develop with similar characteristics. These can develop in the skin without any intensity from the sun, but also the sun's ultraviolet rays can cause these.

Now another characteristic particularly of the melanoma is that it does occur and can occur in light-skinned white people. What happens is if they get too much sun, their skin can blister, get red, and it doesn't heal very fast. This is a sign basically, exposure to the sun's rays by people of light skin. As you come closer to the equator, you find that there's less skin cancer because you're getting closer to dark people or Asian people, the dark people or Africans.

But it is noticed with others who have white skin, blue eyes, red or blonde hair. They are very susceptible to getting a skin cancer with overexposure or regular exposure to the sun. Now, to avoid this, of course, is fundamentally avoiding the sun. And for those that do like the sun, working, playing in the sun, lying the sun, should take precautions, particularly if they're a type of person that's described above and gives a history of family history of skin cancer. All three of these particular skin cancers are treated surgically. That is why I consider them in surgical tips. They can be treated by removal and a general surgeon can do this, a hand surgeon or a dermatologist, because this is technically complicated because the thickness of the lesion determines pretty much the type of treatment and prognosis. That's why I would recommend the dermatologist.

I would also include in the symptoms as described above, the thickening or hardness of the skin lesion. Most of the skin lesions that are normal, soft in texture and feeling, if it seems to be getting harder, the status of the form it takes is very suspicious.

Like all things in the practice of medicine and treatment, the earlier it can be examined, the better the outcome is. So if you have any of the symptoms above and fit in to that type of white skinned person, I advise you to go to your dermatologist as soon as possible. Particularly if you're going to sit in the sun. Among the information you might get from the dermatologist prior to going out into the sun for a vacation or whatever you prefer, ask him or her about any sunscreen you can apply and where you can apply it. I'm not aware of any new protective sunscreen, but it would be a small price to pay to avoid going through one of these types of lesions.

FUTURE OF SURGERY

After you have read this book, you will understand the complications and difficulty and the intensity of the practice of medicine, especially surgery, on the patients. I've taken this opportunity to give future projections of surgery. In other words, what do we see in the future? What are we trying? First is eventually I conclude after years of study and training, that we hope that medication will change the need or the type of surgery. Medical cure, radiation, chemotherapy, whatever it involves, if we can treat the patient perfectly, maybe surgery can be eliminated. This is an important thought in our mind whenever we see patients. This could be in the form of a question to your doctor, "Is the surgery going to be performed open or closed?" Open is when they open an incision and make the incision as such the major part of the operation to get what is done. Closed, the scope is to be used. This is extremely important because the open operation has an incision postoperatively that has to heal. All of that takes time. Using the scope, these are just several openings that are small and a major operation can be done through this, eliminating the big incisions, which take the time to heal. Now, it should be mentioned that the surgeon may say to you it'll be the scope or closed; however, if there's anything that comes up, more visualization, bleeding, et cetera, the surgeon will immediately convert this to an open operation, which is perfectly indicated and should be done.

In the future, it would be a wonderful situation where the surgery would be limited to trauma and organ transplants and plastic surgery so that the other type of surgery, general surgery, could be treated with medication, radiation, et cetera. That is our goal in our research and study of not only how to do the surgery better with less complication and less problems to consider elimination of the need for surgery and treatment of the problem with medication. Only time will tell of this progress, but I have full confidence in the state and practice of medicine to solve the problem by the highly trained, intelligent, efficient doctor's doing this.

Please note that Fellow of the American College of Surgery identifies that the MD or DO is a board certified trained surgeon. You can easily know this. When you go in the doctor's office, he will have the plaque or picture of his diploma that states he has had the appropriate training, and of course ask him/her.

I should also include that it would be very good for the patients and doctors if most of the surgery or type of surgery could be done through the laparoscope. It would be less complication, less recurrence of the problem, and just much easier to go through surgery and the postoperative care.

Respectfully submitted,
John D Sanidas, MD, F.A.C.S.(Fellow of the American College of Surgery)

ABBREVIATIONS YOU SHOULD KNOW

In this age, we have various ways of distinguishing the people who are taking care of us, and most of it is done with a medallion, or identification card, or even in a emblem or what have you. But the main abbreviations, you should know all the following:

MD - means Doctor of Medicine.

DO - means Doctor of Osteopathy. (There is little difference between the two.)

RN - is a Registered Nurse. He/She has taken the training and has passed his or her examination and license to work as a nurse.

LPN - equals a Licensed Practicing Nurse. These nurses have sufficient nurse training to take care of patients. He/She is slightly under the Registered Nurse.

PA - stands for Physician Assistant. It's just exactly what the person does, and it is necessary to have special medical training.

NP - this signifies that this nurse is a Nurse Practitioner. He/She is well trained in the practice of medicine, and in certain areas they can practice without a physician, and in certain areas they must be under the supervision of a physician, depending on the status of licensing by the state.

All the above are involved in the teaching and caring for patients, both in the medical office or hospital.

FACS - Fellow of the American College of Surgery. Signifies that the doctor is fully trained in surgery.

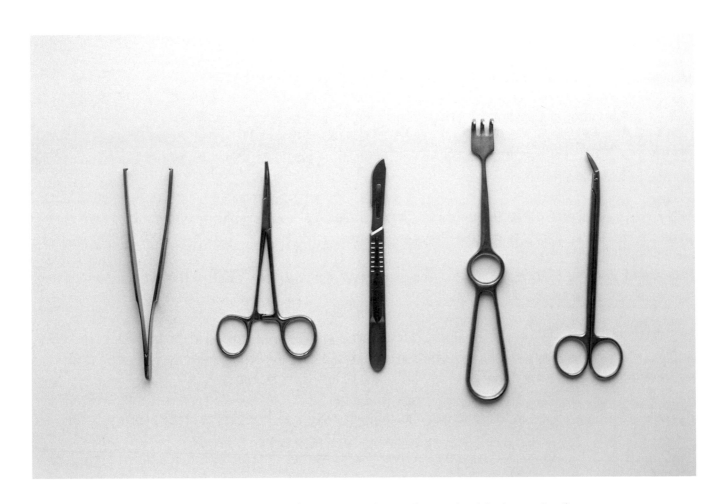

Surgical Instruments (tweezers, pliers, clamp the blade, scalpel)

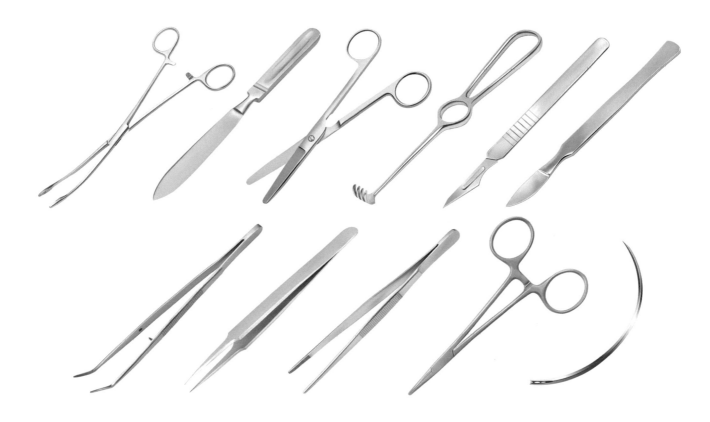

Set of surgical instruments. Different types of tweezers, scalpels, Liston s amputation knife, clip with fastener, straight scissors, Folkmanns jagged hook, Meyers forceps, surgical needle.

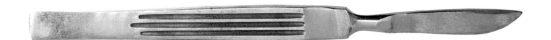

Old Medical Scalpel

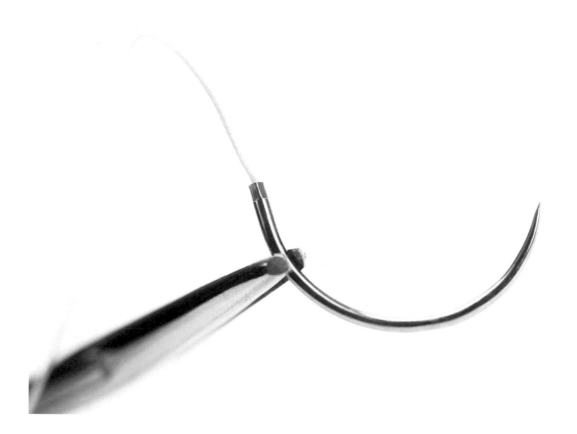

Suture Set

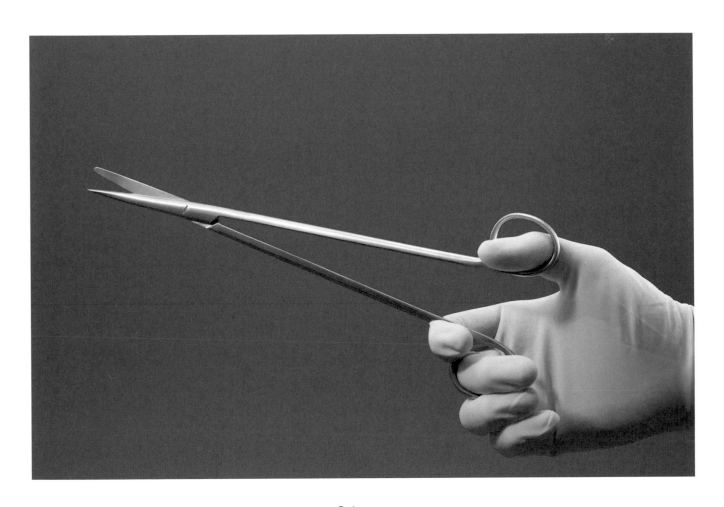

Scissors

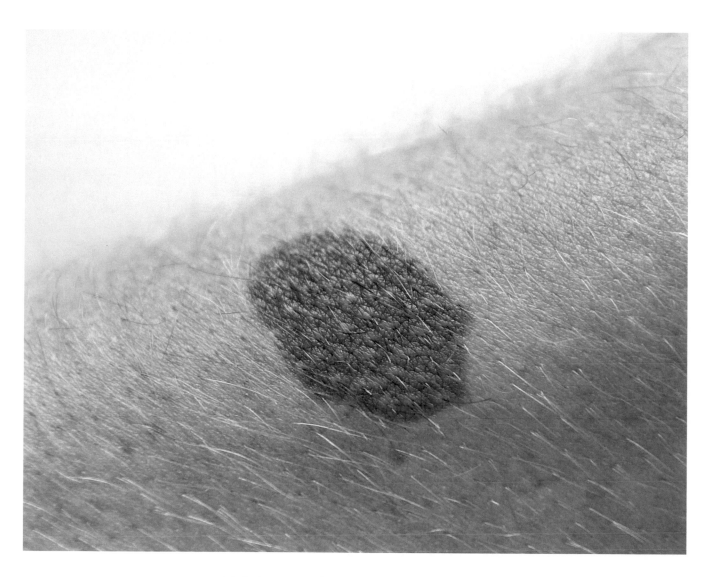

Mole liver spot birthmark on human skin

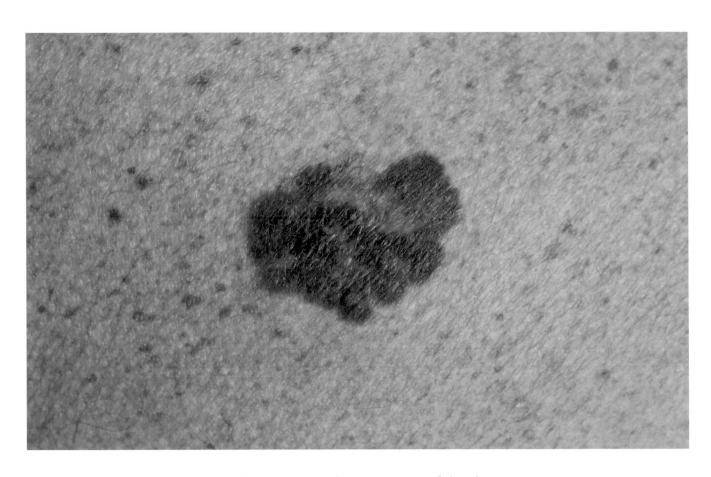

Melanoma - a malignant tumor of the skin

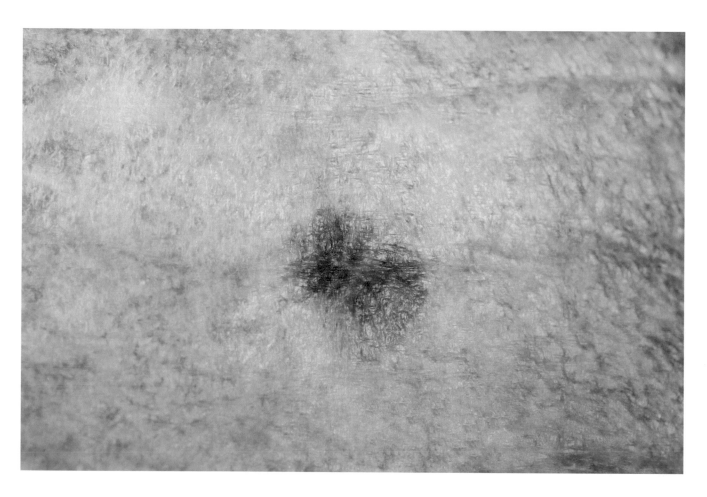

Lentigo Maligna Melanoma on a mans forehead after a biopsy. There
are two stitches holding the biopsy site together.

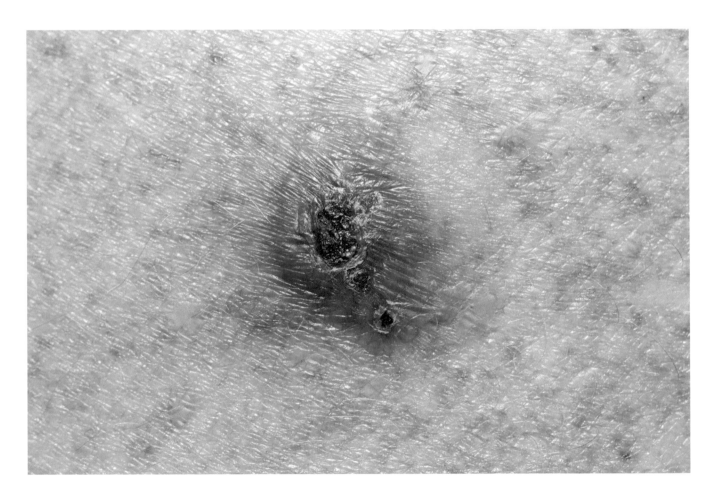

Basal Cell Carcinoma

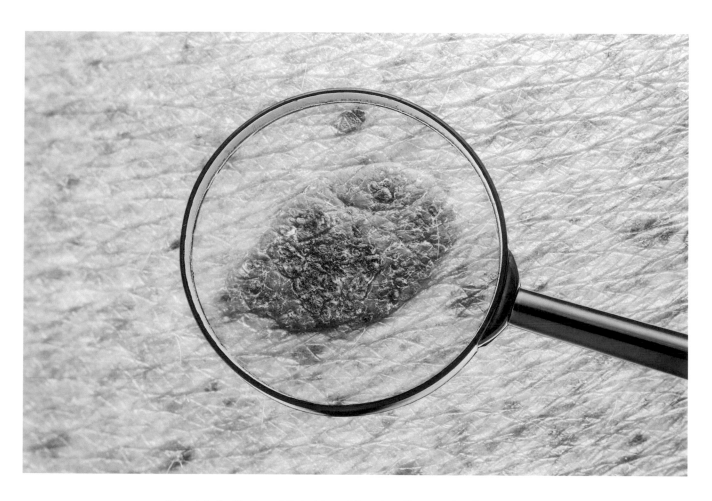

Skin Mole Defect High Magnification for Medical Diagnosis

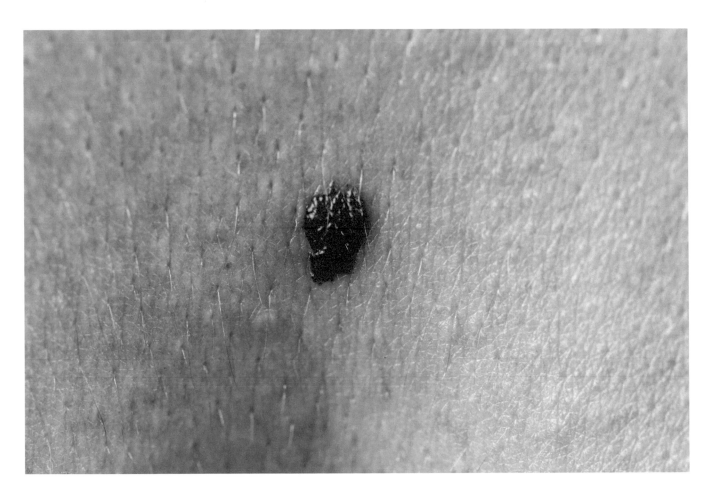

Dangerous mole, sign for skin cancer.

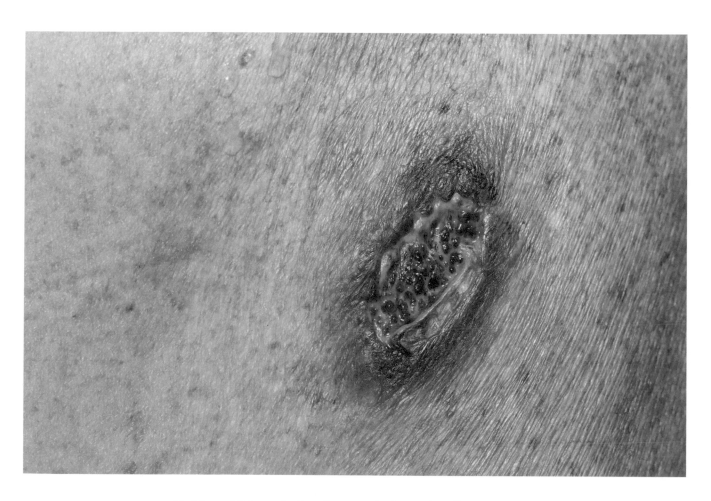

Dehisced Wound after Removal of Basal Cell Carcinoma

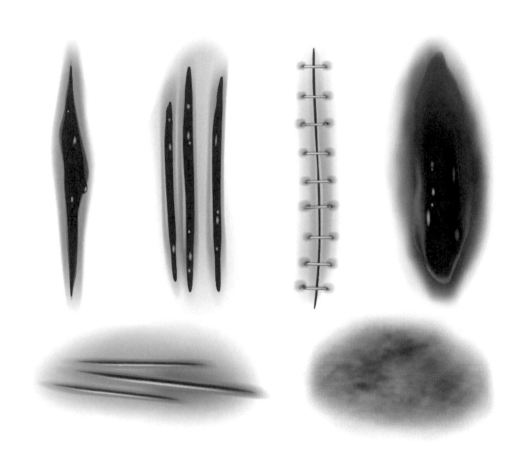

Realistic scars, cuts, wounds, bruises, stitches

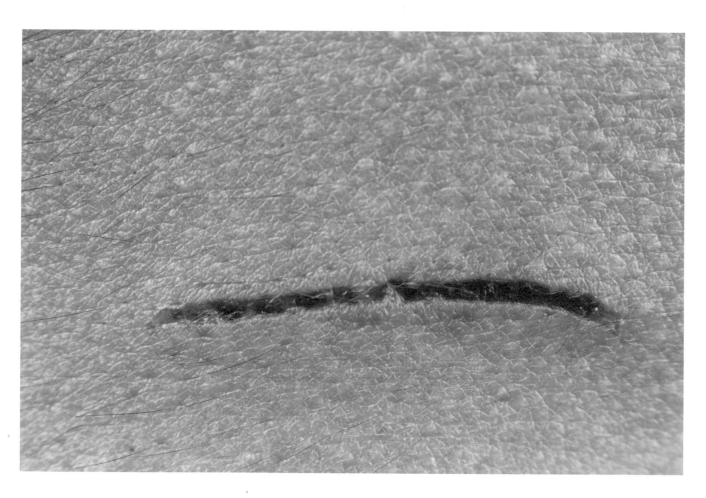

Close up of painful wound on forehead from deep cut

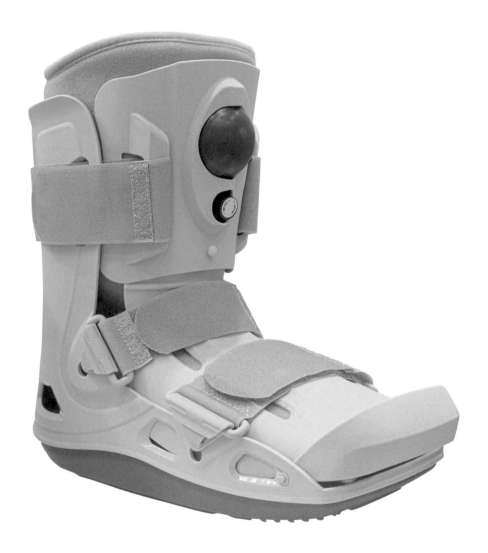

Soft cast right ankle boot for adult, soft cast legs and ankle cover type that designed for patients with orthopedic surgery injuries, fracture and ankle sprain

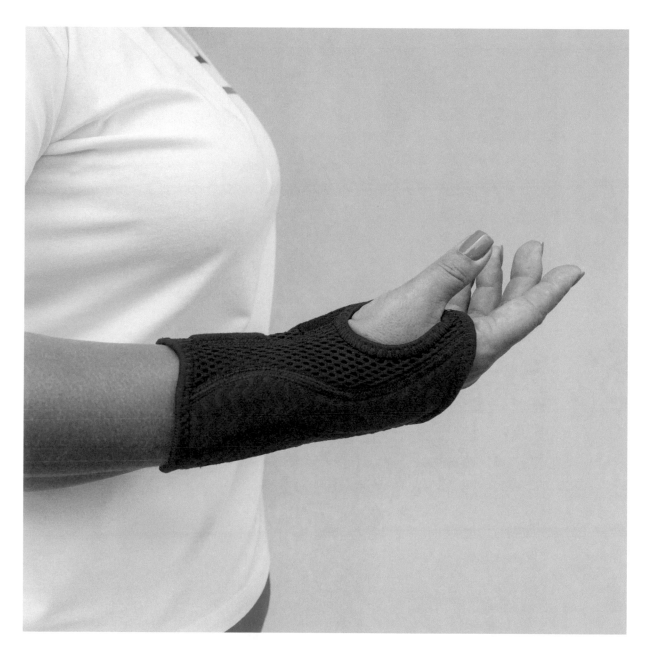

Black wrist brace or corset is worn on women's hand for treatment of carpal tunnel syndrome or median nerve compression, numbness hand

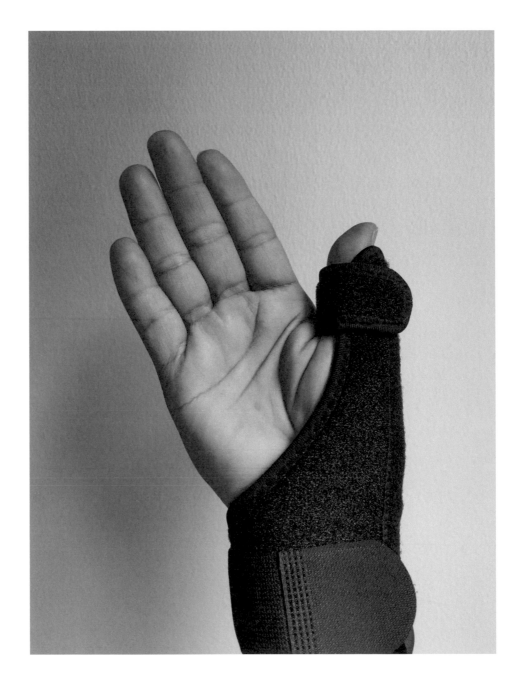

Hand and wrist in a brace

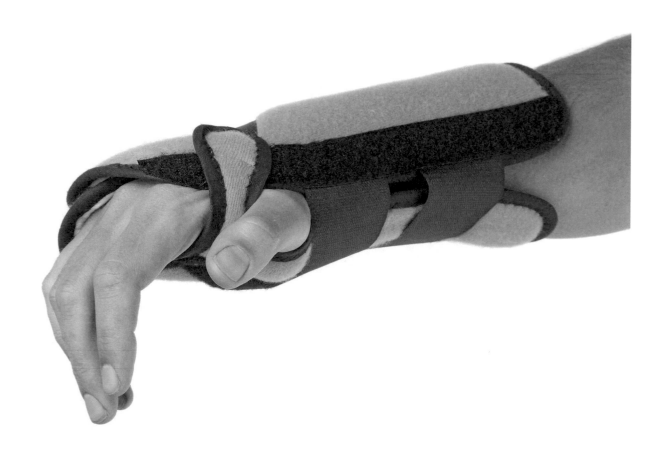

Human arm with wrist brace

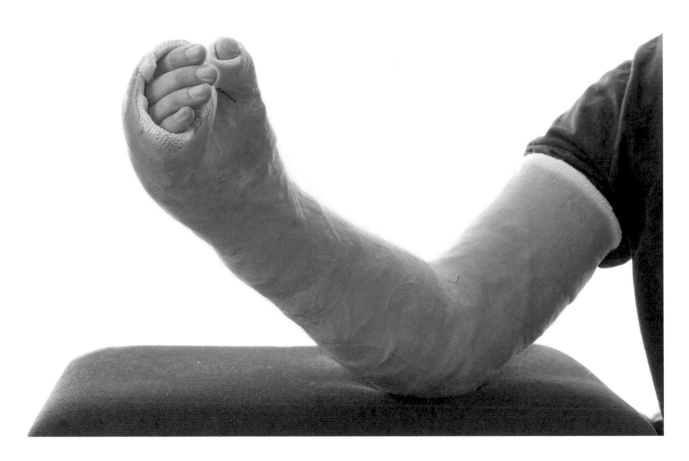

Cast on a human arm

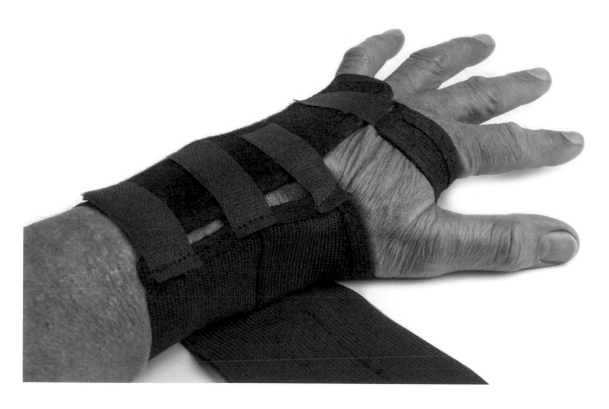

Black hand splint

First, Do No Harm.

-Aristotle (Greek Philosopher) 384-322 BC

ABOUT THE AUTHOR

John D. Sanidas, M.D., F.A.C.S., is a retired general and trauma surgeon. He spent nearly four decades practicing surgery. This is a small culmination of what he has learned throughout his career.

Printed in the United States
by Baker & Taylor Publisher Services